WHEN GOOD MEN GET BURNED

WHEN GOOD MEN GET BURNED

How To Cope and Reinvent Yourself as A Divorcee

Kodi BLACKMAN

DEDICATION

To the many men out there,
In whose nature it is to love,
In whose character it is to do good,
You may get burned being good.
But never let the pain win.
Or become what you are not.
Stay good, but stay wise.

CONTENTS

INTRODUCTION

There are no victors in divorce or relationship breakdowns; everybody loses something. Always remember that.

When I got divorced about a decade ago, I didn't know any other divorced people I could reach out to for solace or who could hold my hand through it all. Recognizing the importance, I became a guide to other men who otherwise would have gone through it alone. I have even met men I could have never imagined would be mentioned in the same sentence as *"divorce."*

When divorce happens, you have a choice – live and manage it, or be bitter and shut the world out. The reality, however, is that whether you stop or continue living - the world continues. In the spur of the moment, you look for right and wrong ideals formed from your interactions with the world. But the world doesn't operate on your outlooks or timeframes. It will feel like it is you against the world.

If you have never been through it, no amount of narration can quite get you to understand how it feels.

This book is not about how to fight your legal battles; it is about helping you come out of a divorce as whole as possible. It is about critical things to remember in the heat of it, so you don't come out too damaged and with too many regrets — and there can be many if you let emotions get the better of the situation. It is about letting you know you are not alone and that other men are going through it just like you, but more importantly, that you will be fine.

Men are usually made to look like *demons* during a divorce. Men stay quiet about their ordeals because society demands we *"swallow it like men."* We cannot show pain, we hardly seek help, and we cannot be fallible. So, we live our pains in silence, not even talking among ourselves as men, because society says we mustn't share our experiences of pain, lest we are called weak.

This book shares some of my experiences and the accounts of others in the hope that it helps the thousands, perhaps millions, of men out there suffering in silence and who do not know what to do.

This is to let you see that just because you already have or are going through a divorce or a relationship breakdown doesn't make you a failure. It is also to offer some help by sharing some of the things you can do amid the confusion.

This book is intentionally concise. It has no fluff; it is to the point. It doesn't try to hide emotions behind politically correct texts. That is because your mind works differently when going through an invested relationship breakdown. It is easy for someone not going through it to read this book and disagree with its content, maybe even find it downright offensive. Luckily, it was not written for them. It was written for men who still have much good in them but must face irreparable relationship breakdowns or, ultimately, divorce. Whether your partner initiates it or you do, doesn't matter; the bruises feel the same – painful.

Hopefully, this short book lets you see that many of us have been through what you are going through and that you are neither insane nor alone. No, you are not, and you will be fine; believe me, you will.

Good luck!

CHAPTER ONE

AN OCEAN OF MIXED EMOTIONS

Divorces and invested relationship breakdowns happen in all shapes, shades, and sizes. One thing is sure, though – there will always be that one event that triggers the final descent. Almost like being on a flight, there's always that final announcement by the pilot over the intercom – *"Ladies and gentlemen, we are now on our final descent to Ex international airport..."* or the lights in the cabin dim. All the cabin crew hurriedly take their seats, and you start to feel the plane's altitude drop. Sometimes you feel a *"whoosh"* in your stomach; other times, you don't, but it becomes apparent – *we are going down.*

In the case of Benny, he had assumed he and his now ex-wife were making progress in recovering their marriage when out of the blue, he got a court summons. In the cases of James and Kaykay, they came home to find that their wives had disappeared with their children. In the cases of Jayden, Bobby, Paul, and Samuel, the final descent happened when the police and social service officers appeared on their doorsteps. For Kofi and Xavi, the last bells rang when they realized their families' joint bank accounts had been emptied while they were away traveling on business... the list is endless. And whether it happens slowly or suddenly, every man will remember the point at which their *"final descent"* announcement was made. When that final realization dawns, the point at which it becomes crystal clear your marriage is over, the point at which you know, *"OK, there's no turning back now"* – irrespective of whether you initiated the divorce or the final call for separation or not, that's when you feel yourself drowning in an ocean of mixed emotions.

No book or song can ever quite capture how many emotions you are swarmed with at once, how long each lasts, or which is most intense. Honestly, in that state, you don't give a freaking fuck – you just go through it all, second after second, minute after minute, day after day, then week after week. You probably have never felt that way before, and I doubt you will ever feel that way again.

You will feel LOW! And as logical as men are, the first question is usually, "*What happened?*" And especially if you are broadly considered a "*good man*," I mean, when you haven't done or been doing any of the typical things known to increase the risk of marital breakdowns – i.e., generally, you haven't been womanizing, abusing your wife, maltreating your children, excessively drinking. Let's say you have been primarily responsible, done your best to put the family first, etc... The sunken lowliness feels even heavier, and the questions, "*What happened? What did I do wrong?*" get even more poignant.

Next, you will feel shocked. When my ex-work colleague, Carlos, called me after coming home to an empty house and finding a divorce court summons and a letter from his then-wife – for days, he remained in a state of stupor. No, he wasn't acting; he genuinely was shocked at how quickly things had escalated. For almost a week, he refused to believe what had happened, refused to accept that the letters and court summons were real, refused to believe his wife and two kids were gone, and ultimately refused to believe his marriage was over. Alfred, our mutual friend, and I became his guardians for a few weeks and had to slap him out of his stupendous shock metaphorically. So, if you are going through this or already have – know that it is normal.

I am not a psychologist, so I haven't done any scientific research on why men initially feel this heavy lowliness and shock. Still, I hazard the theory that, with men, escalation is a function of our logic. In other words, we tend to gauge the timing and intensity of escalations or deteriorations in our relationships devoid of emotions *(feelings)* and primarily based on whether the risks or evidence available reasonably justifies the escalation or deterioration level. When an escalation or deterioration materializes at a particular time or at a certain level of intensity that, in a man's mind, existing risks and evidence do not support – yes, shock ensues. Mentally first, then in every other way next. It's why you will hear a man say things like, *"Did it have to come to this?"* or, more often, *"Was that really necessary?"* Because, in our minds, the timing and intensity of an action may have been premature compared to the risk or evidence that supports the escalation.

Guys, you need to understand that most women are, first and foremost, emotional beings. Their first instinct is NOT to go through a *risk-evidence-escalation* matrix or logical profiling process to determine when an escalated action is justified and at what level of intensity. They act based on how they feel. Feelings can happen, and when they do, most women tend to act on them much more readily than men will. It doesn't mean men don't.

Logical profiling, on the other hand, requires some time to process, which is often the reason for the timing differences in actions between men and women. I am not saying all these things are definite for every man and every woman – these are my studious observations. If the feeling is intense, you can guarantee the intensity of the resulting actions will be too.

Jared and Sophia are both terrific friends of mine. When they realized their marriage was crumbling, they each independently and at different times asked for my advice. Without mincing words, I told them both they needed to see a psychologist for some counseling – and they did. After several sessions, a few unpleasant truths came up. But that was to be expected; it is the nature of these kinds of exercises – everything comes out on the table, and both parties can see what the way forward should be more clearly.

Interestingly, the discoveries came up with things about Sophia that Jared was only getting to know for the first time. I raise this because if anyone was remotely even entitled to be *"angry,"* it should have been him. Logically, however, he considered that getting all these things out on the table was necessary for healing their relationship and, thus, was willing to see it through. And we all believed that was the case. The following week, however, at a Wednesday evening counseling session, Sophia presented her legal divorce papers to Jared and their counselor. Not at the beginning of the session, not at the end of it – in the middle. Naturally, Jared's logic swung into motion – *"Why now? Why in the middle of a joint effort?"* He couldn't understand it all. Logically, his shock and frustration made sense – filing for divorce doesn't just take a fifteen-minute walk to a lawyer's office on the way to a counseling session. Right? So, unsurprisingly, Jared started wondering if Sophia had been planning her divorce proceedings the entire time she attended the sessions with him. If you think about it, Sophia may have acted on her feelings about the marriage long before the counseling sessions commenced or in its early stages. Jared was going through with the process because, logically, the risks and physical evidence *(i.e., mutual attendance by both parties)* did not at that stage warrant the marriage heading for an irreversible breakdown.

I have come to accept that one of the mysteries of marriage is that the very day you agree to live with someone happily forever is the same day you inherently also sign up for the possibility that, at some point in that journey, their happiness may require that you are not *"in the picture."* If you can accept that from the get-go, little will surprise you at any time in the future of that relationship – marital or not. Here is the unpleasant truth: whether we realize it or not, our happiness doesn't depend on anybody else but ourselves. We make the mistake of allowing our happiness to become a function of someone else's presence in our lives. And when one of the parties reverts to their default setting of not *needing another person to be happy*, the other party gets hurt, sometimes badly. We should all go into relationships and marriages with this mindset so that, as long as *YOU are present*, you should be happy. If it must take another person's presence to be happy, you might be emotionally enslaved.

Well, for now, you are divorced, divorcing, separated, or your relationship has suddenly broken beyond repair. You are drowning in a surge of unpleasant emotions and their every derivative – anger, sadness, fear, disgust, hopelessness, betrayal, misery, loneliness, anxiety, stress, desperation, confusion, irritation, hurt, vengeance, frustration, bitterness, emptiness… and on and on and on.

It's normal to feel disoriented, and naturally, the first thing most men do is to try and re-live the last everyday experiences they had become used to with their partner. Sooner or later, you will realize your partner isn't there – physically or emotionally, so the scenarios you are re-living don't exist. Yes, as painful as it is to be jolted back into facing your new reality, you must. She's done with you, or you are done with her.

It takes a while to sink in, but it will. For now, there are a million unanswered questions. You will try to trace your mind back to possible causative scenarios you may have missed. Did it play out slowly, and you refused to see it? Or was it, in fact, a tsunami that just hit you out of the blue, and you couldn't have seen it coming? Yes, that's you amid everything, trying to establish whether you were just naive or your shock is justified. And why not? An emotional turmoil this *"fucked up"* had to have started from somewhere. Don't worry; your sense of *"man-logic"* has no beginning or end. It runs endlessly.

When a marriage breakdown happens, you will feel your world caving in. You will feel you have been made to stand in the middle of a big hole while helplessly buried under the sand. You will feel you are the only one this is happening to. But you will start to realize that you are not the only one. Sooner or later, you will find out other men are going through it from all walks of life. Yep, it almost feels like a private men's club, whose members you only get to know after you have been fully *"inducted."* If you think about it, it's not too surprising – men, for generations, have been primed by society to *"swallow their problems like men"* – so really, who will they talk to about experiences like these? Why would you talk about something that makes you feel like a failure per society's programming?

When my breakdown happened, I had to temporarily move out of our house to live in another part of town. I had to order packaging boxes at my new temporary place to store a few items as I didn't need everything then. It turns out that the gentleman who delivered the boxes was someone I knew – Femi. He was surprised to see me, and in his innocence, his first question was, *"Oh, has the family moved here now?"* To which I sheepishly shook my head and managed to blurt out a weak, *"No, just a temporary thing for me."* He paused before responding, *"Woman issues, huh?"* I didn't know whether to be surprised or grateful that he understood where I stood at my emotional crossroad. Is *"woman issues"* so obviously written on my face? I pondered quietly.

Well, suffice it to say, two hours and two rounds of coffee later, Femi had narrated to me his ordeal. I was gobsmacked. All the while he was going through his narration, I kept thinking, *'You too?'* Yes, well, him too, you too, me too. And you will eventually discover that many others are either going through it too, have been, or will in the future. And if it is any consolation, then know this – you are not alone in this, and bro, welcome to the academy; you are not a failure.

At this point, your highest priority is your mental health – you need to put yourself first. You must do whatever is necessary to calm your mind from the emotional rollercoaster so that you can face the long journey ahead. You need it for you, and if you have kids, for them too. I don't care what you must do to get that done, but it is the most critical thing at that point – your sanity, your calm mind. Check-in with a friend with a *"big ear and an even bigger heart"* who can give you the space to reel your mind in from running wild, get a massage to ease your nerves, take an ice bath if that helps, go for an underwater swim in a good pool, binge on some stand-up comedies, smoke a cigar… do whatever is necessary and reasonable to calm your mind without putting yourself at further risk of emotional or physical harm.

You need a steady, strong, and sharp mind to get through the weeks and months ahead – you need YOU, now more than ever.

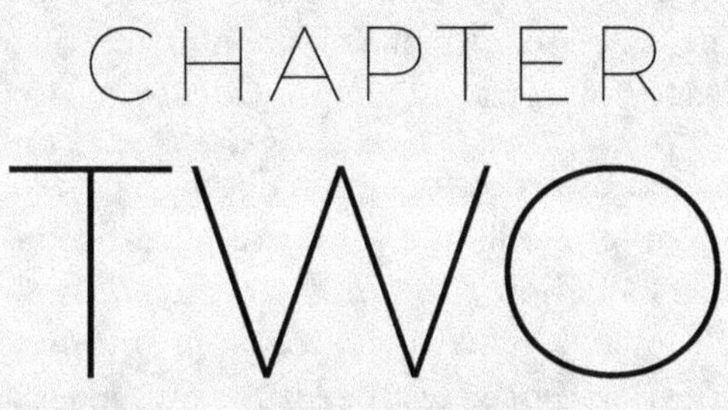

HAVE YOU SEEN AN ANGRY BIRD BEFORE?

You are going to be angry. No, you are going to be fucking furious.

And it is normal. You probably haven't been this angry and confused all at once, and I want you to know you are not going mad. A little stressed from it all, maybe, but not insane. You are normal, you are human, you are not the first, and you certainly, are not alone.

I have been divorced for over a decade, and even writing this chapter swells me with a residual bit of anger. So, I understand how you feel if you are just now going through it or if it hasn't been too long since you went through it. I am not here to explain your anger away; I am just trying to let you know it is OK to be angry and hopefully to help you understand why you have this anger and what you can do to get through it.

Everyone's divorce initiation event is different. Sometimes it crawls in, and you can see it coming. Other times, it comes with a big bang. Quite honestly, even if you saw it creeping up on you, there is a 90 percent chance you brushed it aside, wrote it off because you either didn't expect that from your partner or didn't want to think about her like that, and rightfully so – you trust her, for goodness' sake, she is *(or was)* your partner.

My Ex-wife demanded my passport, our children's birth certificates *(I was a meticulous keeper of our family documents)*, and a sponsorship letter from me to help her apply for her citizenship. It was weird because it was all so sudden, so pressured, and so intense. And here is why it felt that way – I had been trying to get my Ex-wife to file her application for European citizenship for two straight years prior. She had the right to remain in Europe but hadn't been bothered about being officially recognized as a citizen or getting a passport. So, you can imagine how I felt when suddenly, within the space of a week, she had brought her sister over, stayed up late overnight for two days to fill out her forms, pressured me for documents, put supporting documents together, had an express delivery of her application to the Government Bureau, and paid for it from resources hurriedly wired from her family overseas, even though I had offered in the past to take care of it all. And despite all the weird feelings about it, the frantic nature of it all… I still convinced myself, *"Come on, Kodi, this is your wife. She just feels this is the right time to get it done."*

A few days after her application was made, I went to pick up our kids from school as usual, and… they had been collected – and that is how it all blew up – she never returned home, nor did our children. Was that the only sign? No. Before we got to this point, she had on three occasions threatened divorce, each over the most trivial disagreements. And the point I want to make in all this is, even if it crept up on you, and you still didn't see it coming, you did the right thing trusting your partner and not thinking wrong of her – that's what good men do.

And that, gentlemen, is why you will feel outraged – because you feel you genuinely put 100 percent of your emotions, mind, body, and spirit into your marriage *(or relationship)*, only to be defrauded. Yes – that's precisely how it feels. You feel emotionally defrauded and, in the case of some friends of mine, financially scammed. Don't get me wrong. As good men, you don't invest your emotions, finances, and physical exertions into your marriages in the hope of getting paid back. No, you do so because you believe it is the right thing to do and because your women deserve that.

The feeling of being defrauded crystallizes because you suddenly realize you had been pouring and investing your emotions, strengths, and finances into someone who didn't deserve it – emotions, energies, and finances you will never get back. You feel like you were pouring out everything you had in you, just as you would fuel into a vehicle *(the "family"),* in the hope that it will carry you all over the long distance into old age, only to find out that your co-driver had truncated the journey and left you stranded in the middle of the road, most times driving away with the car, or sometimes, leaving the vehicle, but with no fuel in it. The anger can be intense because this is someone you very likely wouldn't have left stranded in the middle of the journey, empty and alone. Yes, you will feel betrayed.

Very soon, even her voice irritates you profusely, her name irritates you, just seeing her irritates you. When her calls or text messages pop up on your phone, your heart rate doubles, and anger rises within you. Everything and anything about her irritates you – her friends, her school-mates, her family, the food she liked, the places she loved to hang out at. It can be so intense that, in some cases, I have had friends say to me that any woman they see during that period irritates them. At some point in all that anger, you may even feel the need to pay her back, punish her, or something. Yes, you will feel like this is an injustice done to you, and she cannot go scot-free. You desperately want to expose her for whom you think she is. I know how it all feels.

But I'll say this to you – DON'T. Please, DON'T do it.

You got here because you were good to someone who didn't appreciate your value in her life. So, take a deep breath and answer this – "*Are you angry at her for showing you her true colors or at yourself for being a good person to her?*" The answer is that you cannot now start wishing you were a bad person, no bro, that's not you, and you certainly cannot allow someone to turn you into something you are not. If that happened, she would have won, and you lost.

Listen, man, I was angry for two straight years, but I never wanted to become an evil, mean person to her, to other women, or to anyone for that matter, simply because one human on a planet of over 8 billion humans, failed to appreciate the good man that I am. It is in your nature to be good. They may have lost you, but you shouldn't lose who you are, too – that would be worse than the betrayal and fraud you feel *(or felt)*.

The decision not to go out there and drag yourself in the gutter for the sake of hurting her, exposing her, or serving her your version of deserving justice, does not mean the pain and anger will vanish into thin air. It means you are justifiably angry BUT, remarkably, smart enough not to become the person who caused you the pain.

I like to be honest; I would be a hypocrite to immediately say to you, *"You have to forgive her; it is for your own good to forgive her… bla bla bla"*— that's a truckload of nonsense. You have to be angry. It would be best if you let out the pain. Then, forgiveness will come when that painful energy has been released. It could be in days, weeks, months, or even years. But if you allow yourself to heal, it will come.

You will repeatedly replay possible *"WHYs"* in your mind, trying to find logical answers to why what happened did, because often, your Ex won't explain the real reason behind her actions. You will also replay countless versions of *"WHAT,"* trying to figure out what you may have done to trigger the breakdown. And yes, your mind will often replay the "WHEN," trying to figure out when it started building up to the breakdown point.

I spent days trying to play back events, even going back to a time before we got married, to see if I missed a timeframe of events I shouldn't have missed. All through this, your brain is looking for a logical answer to the question, *"WHY did this happen?"* The frustration left by replaying these gaps fuels the anger even more.

We, men, are mainly logical, and women are primarily emotional. It would be best to accept that you cannot logically comprehend emotions and, for that matter, decisions, and actions based on those emotions. Sorry to break it to you, but for your own sanity and mental health, you must accept that you may never get a logical answer to the WHY — at least not from her, most likely. If we can understand that *"life"* is good at some things and bad at others and that if we are going to be successful at living it, we ought to embrace its dual nature. Then we will have made significant progress in dealing with our anger during the harsh periods of divorces or family breakdowns. Life is good at "*happening*" and terrible at "*explaining why it happens.*"

In the next chapter, I will share a text exchange I had with my good friend Kenny, seven weeks into hearing for the first time *(through receiving a court summon)* that his wife, Bea, was seeking a divorce. It captures an honest and raw conversation with a good man, unfiltered during a divorce journey. I have only taken out the dates. You may identify with some of it, or you may not, but you will at least get a sense that you are not alone in this dark lonely period of your life.

The singular advice I wish to give you on being angry is summed up at the end of the next chapter. Keep reading.

CHAPTER
THREE

BRO, IT'S KENNY. GOT A MINUTE?

8:42 p.m. - Kenny: Bro, the disappointment is turning into severe anger, disgust, and resentment.

8:42 p.m. - Kenny: Did you go through the same?....

9:24 p.m. - Blackie: *Bro, sorry, was on Zoom. Yeah, I did man. I did. I feel what you feel man. It's understandable. You feel like you poured in your energy and got emotionally defrauded in the process.*

9:24 p.m. - Blackie: *But look at it this way, bruh…*

9:26 p.m. - Blackie: *You did your part - clean, fair, and diligently. No one, not even her or the kids can point a finger at you for lack of trying. In the end, it's her loss, not yours*

9:26 p.m. - Kenny: I feel like I was defrauded.

9:26 p.m. - Blackie: *Yep!*

9:27 p.m. - Kenny: But bruv, the way I'm feeling, if I'm not guarded, I will get vindictive with this whole divorce and destroy her. I'm really pissed off. Seething anger. The kind that's simmering if you know what I mean.

9:27 p.m. - Kenny: It's rough.

9:29 p.m. - Kenny: You know how they say the quiet ones when provoked are more dangerous than the ones that make noise?

9:30 p.m. - Blackie: *I do.*

9:30 p.m. - Blackie: *That's not you, bruh!*

9:31 p.m. - Kenny: It's the old me, man, and I can feel it's trying to come back. I am fighting an inner battle here my guy. kmt.

9:32 p.m. - Blackie: *Interestingly, a part of you knows deep down that you are a good man. You are. But you mustn't let her actions turn you into something you are not. Please.*

9:32 p.m. - Blackie: *Do it for the kids.*

9:33 p.m. - Blackie: *Do it for you. You should win this. Emotions in times like this try to bring out things that make us look just like the frauds we are dealing with. Don't let that win!*

9:33 p.m. - Blackie: *Trust me, you'll regret it knowing she won the ultimate war of making you something you aren't!*

9:34 p.m. - Kenny: But such acts and behavior cannot go unpunished. She is taking the ultimate piss.

9:35 p.m. - Blackie: *No, she is just being herself. Here is the thing, bruh... A snake will always be a snake- whether a pet or in the wild - it bites.*

9:37 p.m. - Blackie: *You, wanting to punish her is not you seeking justice. What you are doing is allowing right and wrong to win over being true to yourself.... if you are true to yourself, you will say you are a good, not a vindictive man. Kings rule with their heads, not hearts. You need to beat the emotions and STAY true to you - a good man.*

9:38 p.m. - Blackie: *That is the biggest WIN man - that despite it all, you never lowered yourself to becoming something you are not.*

9:38 p.m. - Kenny: Mtcheeeew. kmt

9:38 p.m. - Blackie: *Check this out…*

9:38 p.m. - Blackie: *Something I learnt much later…*

9:38 p.m. - Blackie: *Bruv, it takes the Greater to forgive the Lesser.*

9:39 p.m. - Kenny: Mtchew. Fuck that, man!

9:39 p.m. - Blackie: *You know it's true, man. Tell me it isn't.*

9:40 p.m. - Kenny: Snakes need their heads crushed, no? It's Biblical.

9:40 p.m. - Blackie: *Crushing the serpents head was meant for an attack on the leadership of David's -lineage – Jesus.*

9:41 p.m. - Blackie: *K, you know Karma is a BLAATCH right?*

9:41 p.m. - Kenny: I like to create my own karma. Grin.

9:41 p.m. - Kenny: People like that don't learn until they are taught a bitter lesson on reality.

9:41 p.m. - Blackie: *You just want something to justify your anger.*

9:43 p.m. - Blackie: *Why? Are you Grandmother Karma or Grandmama Bitch?*

9:44 p.m. - Blackie: *Bro, make God proud. Let Him do the retaliation. "Vengeance is mine sayeth the Lord" right?*

9:44 p.m. - Kenny: That's your translation. Mine is different lol.

9:44 p.m. - Blackie: *fuck you bro lol!!!*

9:45 p.m. - Kenny: If God was serious about vengeance, Mr. Z would have lost the last election man

9:45 p.m. - Blackie: *We don't always see God's ways bro. What if He let Z win to get citizens to feel the price of voting foolishly last election*

9:46 p.m. - Blackie: *let***

9:46 p.m. - Kenny: Foolish people don't learn. Proverbs.

9:46 p.m. - Kenny: So what will they really learn? Noffin'!!!!!.

9:47 p.m. - Blackie: *They don't learn IF you try to instruct them. They learn by Going through PAIN, which is the classroom for those who choose not to learn as sensible people do.*

9:48 p.m. - Kenny: Mtchew. Fuck your philosophical talk man. I want ACTION

9:49 p.m. - Kenny: Hahah!

9:51 p.m. - Kenny: My friend, you're changing the topic of discussion here. Pussy!

9:51 p.m. - Blackie: *Hahahahaha! You need some sexual healing too bruh lol. Shall I go call you Bea?*

9:52 p.m. - Blackie: *You could do with some spanking. Hahahaha*

9:52 p.m. - Kenny: Hehehe!! Fuck you 1 trillion times man. Fuck you and fuck Bea.

9:52 p.m. - Kenny: Been holding back family members. Think I will just start unleashing them at her

9:52 p.m. - Blackie: *For fuck's sake. Really? Hahahahaha, fucking Hooligan!*

9:53 p.m. - Kenny: I'm serious Lol.

9:53 p.m. - Kenny: I am wasting too much of my energy trying to cool them off.

9:53 p.m. - Kenny: I should get them to go vent on her a bit.

9:53 p.m. - Blackie: *Seriously though, to what end? Everyone is just going thru emotions right now.*

9:53 p.m. - Kenny: Hehehehe!

9:54 p.m. - Kenny: Cos that's what she likes, right? I gave her a fabulous life, she didn't like it, might as well serve her chilli HOT!!

9:54 p.m. - Kenny: Grin.

9:54 p.m. - Blackie: *It is you who needs to say to them, this was your marriage, it was your legacy - this is NOT how you want it painted. Tell them.*

9:54 p.m. - Kenny: I want her foolishness to be properly scrutinized and seen by all.

9:54 p.m. - Blackie: *Prick! What does that fucking make you who married her? Fuck that man. This can't be you talking, bruh!*

9:55 p.m. - Blackie: *You have maintained a brilliant record with Bea and the kids. Don't let family taint it - not your side. It takes two to tango man — so she left the marriage as the 'bad nut,' so what? You also want to turn around and be a bloody bad nut? Are you freaking kidding me?*

9:55 p.m. - Blackie: *Not your business.*

9:55 p.m. - Kenny: Then maybe I should release her dirty info to her godmother and church folks. She is not the saint they think she is

9:55 p.m. - Blackie: *And doing all that makes you an angel with sun-kissed wings, right?*

9:55 p.m. - Blackie: *Raise the bar, man. Raise the bloody bar*

9:55 p.m. - Kenny: She is still going to their fucking choir practice like a Saint.

9:55 p.m. - Kenny: Fuckwit!

9:55 p.m. - Blackie: *Dickhead…*

9:56 p.m. - Blackie: *Even I don't know you to say to you anymore*

9:56 p.m. - Kenny: Lmao. Good

9:56 p.m. - Blackie: *I did some of that vindictive shit out of pure pain and anger. I regret doing it. Don't do it, bruh. Trust me, it will bite you at some point*

9:57 p.m. - Kenny: Then I might even tag her friends and Facebook pals.

9:58 p.m. - Blackie: *Bombocladt! That's not a leaf you want your kids to read about you in the biography that your good nature has written on their minds so far.*

9:58 p.m. - Blackie: *You have raised them to treat others better than you got treated…*

9:58 p.m. - Blackie: *Keep it that way. Don't let them be disappointed in you too!*

10:00 p.m. - Kenny: Fuck you, man!

10:00 p.m. - Kenny: Are you here to support me or be the voice of TREASON?

10:00 p.m. - Kenny: Fuck off!

10:00 p.m. - Blackie: *I am your bloody Voice of REASON – you can cream your dick with the "T"!*

10:04 p.m. - Kenny: Ha! I hate you man. You are such a fucking bully.

10:04 p.m. - Blackie: *Whatever!! Dude, we can't let them beat us 2 - 0. What I got wrong, you will get right. Period. Where you should fight, I'll ask you to fight. Where you don't need to be vindictive, I will slap you with some sense and tell you not to be vindictive. As for your H-Emotions, there will be fucking lots of it yet to come. It's my job to shred them and burn them whenever I can - they won't do you any good.*

10:05 p.m. - Kenny: Nice speech, but Naaaah! She must suffer the consequences of her foolishness.

10:05 p.m. - Blackie: *It is HER foolishness dude, not yours, so, STOP IT!*

10:06 p.m. - Blackie: *Who made you the nation's moral EXECUTIONER or the moral Hague?*

10:06 p.m. - Kenny: Do you not know you are gods – says the Bible. So, I am sitting in judgement Lol

10:06 p.m. - Blackie: *Madafaakaaaa*

10:07 p.m. - Kenny: Call it righteous anger. The same anger God used to instruct people to be wiped out by the Israelites.

10:08 p.m. - Kenny: You see, the issue with people like that is they have always had their way regardless of their foolishness from childhood. Mollycoddled.

10:09 p.m. - Kenny: So they don't separate the realities and accountability that comes with adulthood from their set behaviors.

10:11 p.m. - Blackie: *Still doesn't make you God's moral sergeant.*

10:12 p.m. - Blackie: *You want to mother and father her now to relearn a better childhood, or you think you would have done a better job than her parents given the same circumstances?*

10:12 p.m. - Kenny: Nah, I want to punish her.

10:12 p.m. - Kenny: Freaking traitor

10:12 p.m. - Kenny: I mean, what a fucking stupid way to betray someone who has been nothing but a blessing. What the fuck did I ever do wrong? I don't drink, smoke, or womanize. What da FUCK!

10:13 p.m. - Kenny: It's fucking dumb though

10:14 p.m. - Kenny: I mean wtf?

10:15 p.m. - Kenny: Jesus, the more I replay the shit the more vexed I get.

10:16 p.m. - Blackie: *This just keeps getting better. Fam, try seeing the humane part of all of this. She may also be going through some mental health issues and not know it, you know? Yo. I know you are angry bro, and that's perfectly fine but dude, can't you see, none of her issues sounds logical? What if she isn't well? You may be angry at someone who doesn't even know she is sick.*

10:16 p.m. - Kenny: *And how is that my problem?*

10:17 p.m. - Blackie: *Yo, breaaathe!*

10:17 p.m. - Kenny: One thing I can't stand is stupidity

10:17 p.m. - Kenny: It gets on my nerves

10:18 p.m. - Blackie: *She is still the mother of your kids. You need her in the equation for your kids, bro.... in as much as you'd wish she was just deleted from your life right now... She will be here for a long time to come. Especially IF the court decides to give her full or shared custody.*

10:19 p.m. - Kenny: That really gets on my nerves.

10:19 p.m. - Kenny: She doesn't do that much for them anyway.

10:19 p.m. - Kenny: Mtchew.

10:19 p.m. - Blackie: *Fucking hell, man, you need some weed now Bro. I swear, you do. LoL. I will order some for you in your favourite grape juice. Hahhahahaha*

10:20 p.m. - Blackie: *She is still their mother.*

10:20 p.m. - Kenny: Like this morning, the first thing she did was get up and go to church, nothing done at home.

10:20 p.m. - Kenny: Absolute foolishness.

10:20 p.m. - Kenny: Pure hypocrisy.

10:20 p.m. - Blackie: *Most religious folks BURY themselves in "CHURCH" once they feel messed up, it's normal. She's probably just feeling lost in all of this too*

10:20 p.m. - Kenny: That's why I want to expose her to her church folks – can't mess up people's lives and just coil back into the holy fold. FUUUUCK me!!!!

10:21 p.m. - Blackie: *Exposing her - is not your freaggiing job, man. She can do that without you*

10:21 p.m. - Kenny: Mtchew

10:21 p.m. - Blackie: *Your job now is to FOCUS on YOU!*

10:22 p.m. - Kenny: That's exactly what I'm doing by exposing her foolishness.

10:22 p.m. - Blackie: *That's a gig for which the payment comes in the form of marks being deducted from your achieve-ments with the family. Is that what you want?*

10:23 p.m. - Blackie: *Still, without her, you'd not have had these lovely, smart kids.* Thought about that?

10:23 p.m. - Kenny: Dude, you even smoke cigars. You are not allowed to advise on God's behalf kmt

10:23 p.m. - Blackie: *Fuck you, dickhead! Lol.*

10:24 p.m. - Blackie: *Nonsense*

10:24 p.m. - Kenny: Clap for her....

10:24 p.m. - Blackie: *Talking about cigars though — even God inhales the incense on the altars LoL*

10:24 p.m. - Kenny: Dunno why you're even giving her a free pass. You are a weakling bro

10:25 p.m. - Kenny: And you went as far as buying her dinner? Fuck you, bro!

10:25 p.m. - Kenny: She fooled you as well.

10:25 p.m. - Kenny: You should demand the food back, hehehehehe!

10:25 p.m. - Kenny: Make her vomit it all. Lol

10:26 p.m. - Blackie: *I was just helping her see what a beautiful network she was about to throw away. Why are you so eager to dig her pit for her? Why? Are you a gravedigger now? Lol*

10:26 p.m. - Kenny: She won't dig it well. I want to help. I'm nice like dat. Grin.

10:27 p.m. - Blackie: *Even Jesus knew what and who Judas the betrayer was, yet, allowed him to be the Treasurer of his ministry - can you believe that?*

10:27 p.m. - Kenny: That is Jesus's fucking business.

10:27 p.m. - Kenny: I wasn't there. lol.

10:27 p.m. - Blackie: *Haa! Fucking Lucifer.*

10:28 p.m. - Blackie: ROFL

10:31 p.m. - Blackie: *The evil is seething underneath your bleeding skin man…. If we don't tame it, you can easily resurrect Judas Iscariot and kill him again. Hahahahaha!*

10:32 p.m. - Kenny: Nah, I will resurrect him and split the cash with him.

10:32 p.m. - Blackie: *Hahahaha! Maybe even introduce him to Crypto.*

10:32 p.m. - Kenny: Hahahahahha!

10:32 p.m. - Blackie: *Man, you need Valium or chamomile tea by your bedside for nights like this. You are struggling with sleep.*

10:33 p.m. - Kenny: I need to smash someone's head in, is what I need. Mtchew

10:37 p.m. - Blackie: *Let's smash in your emotions first.*

10:37 p.m. - Blackie: *You're scaring me, bro!*

10:37 p.m. - Kenny: Oh

10:37 p.m. - Kenny: Lmao

10:38 p.m. - Kenny: What's funny is, she thinks we should be civil about it all.

10:38 p.m. - Kenny: Like, I should just keep condoning the foolishness.

10:38 p.m. - Kenny: I'm sure with the kids she is expecting me to also be the voice of reason, to bring them round to understanding why she's not a twat.

10:38 p.m. - Blackie: *The kids will make up their own minds. If you ask me - they may already have.*

10:38 p.m. - Blackie: *Best approach is…*

10:38 p.m. - Blackie: *Be silent, for now.*

10:39 p.m. - Kenny: She will have the shock of her life.

10:39 p.m. - Blackie: *Keep a distance.*

10:39 p.m. - Blackie: *SILENCE is neither civil nor antagonistic. So, keep your silence before you tell her something and escalate the mess. Keep your calm, man. If you need space, come hang out with me for a few days. In fact, I think you should do that!*

10:40 p.m. - Blackie: *Yep, just stay out of sight.*

10:42 p.m. - Kenny: Her whole being disgusts me.

10:42 p.m. - Kenny: I am just fucking upset

10:44 p.m. - Blackie: *Naaaaa*

10:44 p.m. - Kenny: Naaaa what?

10:44 p.m. - Kenny: Don't think u quite understand the level of anger I feel

10:44 p.m. - Blackie: *You are just angry that you put in all that effort and got nothing in return from her.*

10:45 p.m. - Blackie: *I've been there, man. Held the anger for a year plus*

10:45 p.m. - Blackie: *Seeing her name, pictures, text, call, anything just got me angry*

10:45 p.m. - Kenny: If I see her, I just go craaazy vex.

10:46 p.m. - Blackie: *But in the end, I was messing myself up.*

10:46 p.m. - Blackie: *Yep*

10:46 p.m. - Blackie: *It's a phase. You will get past it.*

10:47 p.m. - Kenny: In fact, it's even started making me hate females in general.

10:47 p.m. - Blackie: *You're lucky, you have me, bro. I had no one around when my shit hit the fan.*

10:47 p.m. - Blackie: *It'll pass*

10:47 p.m. - Blackie: *You'll fight me for saying that BUT, it will pass!*

10:47 p.m. - Kenny: Today, for example, a colleague at work hugged me. Man, I Just stood there motionless. She was like, "hey you're cold today." The look I gave her man…. Lmao

10:48 p.m. - Blackie: *I can relate.*

10:48 p.m. - Kenny: Sure, sure, I will get past it after I've seen and tasted vengeance.

10:49 p.m. - Blackie: *You won't get any FUCKING vengeance, bruh. Go drink have a beer and sleep. We don't do vengeance here, we do crypto LOL*

10:49 p.m. - Kenny: Mtchew

10:49 p.m. - Kenny: It's a good thing I don't drink too much.

10:50 p.m. - Blackie: *You'll need an outlet though!*

10:50 p.m. - Blackie: *I took to cigars and writing articles.*

10:50 p.m. - Kenny: Outlet for what?

10:50 p.m. - Blackie: *And swimming*

10:51 p.m. - Kenny: Mtchew. Not interested.

10:52 p.m. - Kenny: I need a Hitman, Lol

10:53 p.m. - Blackie: *You need a friend with good vibes who won't let you ruin yourself, motherfucker! lol.*

10:53 p.m. - Kenny: Errr, no thanks.

10:54 p.m. - Blackie: *Like you have a freaking choice. That's it. Dude, pack a bag and go to bed. I'm coming for you at 6am, we'll hike up the hill in my hood and you can come stay at mine for a few days until you cool off.*

10:54 p.m. - Blackie: *Leave Bea and the kids to me – I'll tell them I need your help at my end for a few days.*

10:55 p.m. - Blackie: *Take it easy, buddy. See you in a few hours.*

10:55 p.m. - Kenny: Thanks, man. But still, FUCK YOU man!

10:55 p.m. - Blackie: *Yeah yeah Lol, I LOVE YOU TOO, Dickhead*

I want to bring a few lessons from this chat and the previous chapter to your attention. In these circumstances, you will be angry, or if you are reading this to help someone, they will be angry. Very angry. I beg of you, don't simply attempt to shut down or block the*(ir)* anger – play the fool even if you must. It is better that their bitterness should seep out on you, in a controlled manner, than hurtfully at someone else uncontrollably.

Secondly, get a friend you can trust and someone who can give you a safe space to spill over, vent, or psychologically bleed without them being judgmental. In these circumstances, anyone directly family or closely related to your Ex is bound to come across to you as either compromised or in the camp of your Ex. You need a neutral person with whom some relationship already exists - it is critical and necessary to diffuse all the anger you feel. You may want to say or do things you never have before; I hope your confidante lets you, as long as s/he is in the picture, to ensure you don't end up hurting yourself in any way.

If a friend or family cannot offer you the space you need to *"blow over,"* please get professional help. Take a few days at a retreat with resident psychologists or someone trained to give psychological support. Please.

Whatever the case, you need to diffuse – in a safe space. So, find the space *(or person)* and diffuse around them – NOT IN SOLITUDE. Being by yourself is psychologically not the best environment for you in this situation.

Find a safe space, vent, bleed, pour out, curse, blow over, diffuse… and then get back to stable and calm.

FAMILY AND FRIENDS: MANAGING THE GOOD, BAD, AND THE UGLY

When your marriage or long-term relationship collapses, your family will turn up in various ways. Most will likely be biased toward you; as the saying goes, *"blood is thicker than water,"* so naturally, they will take your side unless you seriously screwed up and deserved this. Hard as that may be, most people prefer to feign loyalty than be seen as the *"traitor"* in your time of need.

Some may stand on the fence and say, even if not to your face, *"We told you so,"* and for them, the loose aim is likely to have the temporary gratification from knowing they were right and you were wrong – let them have their interim win, it'll fade away back into loyalty.

Others will be just as numbed and confused as you are and hardly say much – don't mistake their silence to mean they don't care – most likely, they are genuinely grappling with the shock and confusion too.

Then, there will be the rare, very mature, very emotionally intelligent ones among the lot, who will attempt to hear both your side of the story and your Ex-partner's and then seek to find common grounds for meaningful conversations – for example, if you have any, the mental and emotional safety of you and the children. You need to look out for these latter ones immediately and keep them close in your corner. They are likely to be the ones to help you use your head when your emotions want to take over and, equally, the ones to introduce a bit of heart into your thinking when all you want to embrace is emotionless rationality. They will be your balance because of their maturity, emotional stability, or lessons learned from their own experiences. As I have come to find, some of the rare people who play this role in your breakdown times may not even be blood or family, but for your own good, you must see them as such.

That's the easy part.

The more complex elements of family to deal with in times such as these are those that are both angry and overzealous. On the back of it all, they mean well; believe me, they do, but I can also find a few reasons you need to control what roles they play "*on your behalf*" while you get through the breakdown process. You cannot avoid them, like it or not, but you owe it to yourself to manage them.

Yes, I know; as if the crisis you may be going through is not stressful enough, why do you now have to deal with family folks? Well, understand this, whether you expressly ask these overzealous family folk to have con-frontations, fights, or raise hell with your Ex and her family or not, as far as they are concerned, they are doing it on your behalf, they are doing it because they inher-ently believe it is justice of some sort for you, they are doing it because they are convinced they are the only ones "*divinely or self-mandated*" to do it for you. If you mix all that up with the emotional frenzy everyone will be ex-periencing; you will understand why, later in this chapter, I insist you need to manage these family zealots. Sorry, it doesn't matter if they are mom, dad, sister, brother, or very distant cousins or aunts.

First, it is worth accepting that you contributed to the breakdown. It takes two to dance the tango, and it would be naive to think otherwise; *even angels have dirty wings* from time to time, and that's a given. But let's assume for a minute that with all the human errors on your part, you have still managed to, overall, keep a profile as *"a good man"* in your marriage, or better still, let us even assume wildly that you did not play the final escalation trigger or disintegration event – then you should be aiming to keep that *"clean record"* throughout the divorce process. The last thing you want is for a loose family canon painting you and your *"clean record"* in mud. Don't let it.

When Mace and Farida's marriage broke down, through a combination of infidelities and misspending of family funds, Farida, interestingly, was the first to confess that her *"marriage to a beautiful soul"* collapsed because of her recklessness. This isn't simply about labeling who was good and who was terrible at the time of the breakdown, so let's not make it about that – for you, my concern is that you exit with a clean sheet, however pure it was at the time of the breakdown, not worse.

That was the case with Mace until his temperamental younger sister, Mina, a junior military officer, heard about the unpleasant breakdown, got furious *(on behalf of Mace, of course)* about Farida *"treating her brother like shit"* and so, single-handedly, and without the knowledge of Mace, went over to Farida's parent's home *(where Farida was temporarily cooling off)* to, as she put it *"teach her a lesson."*

Sadly, in the confrontation that ensued, Farida's mother got severely injured, and suddenly, everything changed, from a broken-down marriage that was about to get amicably dissolved to a headline case of assault, damage to property, and putting Mace in a bad spotlight. It was no more about him leaving a marriage in which *"he was be-*

ing treated like shit." Suddenly, he and his family were "*the shitty lot*" – all because of one angry, overzealous family member. It's easy to read this and say, "*Nah, none of my family members will act like that,*" but when a confrontation happens, fuelled by emotions, nobody has a freaking clue how fast and how wildly it can deteriorate; it just does. If you didn't make a bad name for yourself in your marriage before it ended, you shouldn't let your family give you one now that it has ended.

The second thing to remember is if you have been married to someone, how long the marriage lasted doesn't matter here. Your relationship with them will form the memories you will take away, and who they were while it lasted will be lessons to last you a lifetime. The memories and lessons will be a mix of good and bad, but they are the only two blocks that build life itself – good and bad. The vital thing to remember as motivation to control your family's bad reaction to the breakdown as best as possible is – that it was YOUR marriage, it is now YOUR memory, and she was YOUR life lesson, not your family's. I'm not saying you shouldn't feel bad about the breakdown; I'm asking you not to taint the memory and lessons you walk away with – angry or not, they are yours, unpleasant or not, they are yours.

Third, if you had children at the time of your breakdown, and they are aged five years or older, they see and know a lot more than you would give them credit for. Your children had an image of you and your Ex while the marriage bloomed. No matter how short-lived, their mental image of you will form their philosophies about what a good man is and who you are. Please don't ruin it by giving a free pass to a family member who carries no responsibility for the lasting image your children will hold of you.

My children were very young when my ex-wife and I split. Many years after my second daughter had turned fourteen and came to spend her holidays with me, I learned from our conversations how she had struggled to reconcile who she knew me as before the split and the many horrible lies she was fed about me while she lived with her mother. In her own words, she *"always knew none of that was true."* Then she recounted how she thought it was unfair that she and her siblings were taken away from me so abruptly when she knew I loved them so much.

The point I want to make here is this – DON'T let anyone ruin the image your kids have of you in the very critical moments of a breakdown because a lot that happens in that high-intensity, high-stakes, highly emotional period will form some of the strongest and lasting memories of who you were and what you stood for. Don't let someone else ruin it.

Fourth and last, and this is just pure, streetwise logic. If family folks think being vicious, inhumane, crazy, and wild toward your Ex and her family in a sensitive time like this is the way to show you their loyalty, then they either had none to start with, are just too emotional, or have no idea what the realities of breakdowns are. They probably only imagine a future without your Ex in your life or that of the kids. That's OK. It is their worldview on the matter. What they do miss, which is a greater reality, is that even though you may not be physically together if you have children or own joint assets, your paths will continue to cross, whether your family folk like it or not, whether you like it or not. More on that later.

Despite their fundamentally good intentions, family members, I mean, and the many crazy and wild *"on your behalf"* reactions you will witness, their actions may not always be about you, well, not consciously. For some, it is also an opportunity to exorcise their own hidden demons – a dislike for your Ex, an experience of a similar nature they were never fully able to get out of their system, a crystallization of their overprotectiveness of you – hey, maybe you are all that is left of true family they can point to. For some, too, it is the only clear shot of a chance to pay back your goodwill toward them. For them, and subconsciously so, doing this dirty work of *"fighting for you"* is a chance to settle a temporary or lifetime of perceived indebtedness to you - as flattering as it all may sound.

I believe I have given you good enough reasons not to let family ruin anything for you. Don't.

So, what do you do?

When my breakdown happened, I knew one of my cousins would likely raise a storm – let's call her *Jasmine*, but I quickly had to question my assumptions. What if it didn't come from her? What if the storm came from my two quiet and unassuming siblings? So, I did what I usually advise most men to do – be the first to break the news to family, ideally in person and, most importantly, with everyone who matters together, if possible. You don't want your message being re-polished and impregnated with biases and emotions before being delivered to those who weren't present. Let everyone in your immediate family and close circle hear it from you as best you can.

An equally critical part of that conversation is letting them know that you want them to respect your wishes and sensitivities and not have any interactions or confrontations with your partner and her family that you haven't expressly sanctioned. And you need to be clear with them what the support you need from them as a family is precisely – from needing a safe space to stay in the interim to needing someone to look after the kids, to someone being there to listen to you rant from time to time if need be, praying for your family, and so on. Be very clear. This helps them see that they are not being shut out and that there are tangible ways you need them to help you in those trying times. Of course, this is all happening as soon as it is clear to you that there is no going back and that you have exhausted all options to reconcile with your partner – at that point, it is what it is.

I have heard people say there are people you should never talk to about the breakdown until *"the show is over"* for fear of their reactions. To that, I say it is a fifty-fifty play. It might work, but it might not work. See, you may do well to keep your thoughts from everyone, but you cannot guarantee others who know won't tell, even if you explicitly asked them to keep it hush — humans are humans. Then they will wonder why they had to hear it from someone else, not you, or why everyone else knew about it but not them. Well, I like to avoid these awkward pitfalls, so I say, figure out who matters, who has been part of your lives together, who was physically, emotionally, financially, and spiritually invested reasonably in your marriage or long-term relationship, sit them down, repeat the announcement of the *"breakdown,"* rinse, dry, and repeat.

You will need to be firm, and whatever conversations ensue from it, put your peace of mind first. I have a reason for saying that. Different family members may have various reasons they may disapprove of the split. Maybe because of their own experiences, others, perhaps they worry it may bring some embarrassment to the larger family. For some, it is against their faith or religion, while others simply like your partner. For any of these reasons, anyone can be strongly motivated to talk you out of the dissolution process, but the choice will be yours. They may have their reasons, but it is you who lived it, and only you can tell if it is best for you to go back or continue in such a relationship and under what new or unchanged conditions. If you need some time to give it a thought, do that, but never be emotionally coerced into making a U-turn to be with someone you once believed you mustn't live with. It must be your decision, by you, for you.

Good luck. I know you will need it.

CHAPTER FIVE

IN THE MATTER OF KIDS VERSUS...

This chapter was by far the hardest to write, and I imagine it will be the most challenging topic for you to deal with, too – if you have kids between you and your Ex. My divorce came with some physical separation from my children, and if that is the case with you, too, you will probably feel the emotions of temporary *"loss"* flooding back when you get through this chapter; it is normal. If you were lucky to retain custody of your children, great, but it is equally possible you will feel some partial loss on their behalf because they do not have the full complement of father-mother parenthood as they used to. Whatever the case, it is a good starting point that you feel something where your children are concerned – it simply means your heart is in a good place where your kids matter.

I use the term *"lucky"* for men who can gain full custody over their children because in *"most"* divorce cases I have come across and indeed a phenomenon you may be familiar with too *(or not)* – in most jurisdictions *(unless the circumstances under which you separated showed your ex-wife in a harmful, grossly irresponsible, or incapable state of mind or ability)* – it is most likely she will win custody of the children. At best, you may get joint custody. It doesn't matter much if you were the most dominant, positive figure in the kids' lives; the starting point for most custody considerations is that the mother is naturally the *better-wired* party for nurturing children.

I share these things so that when you must deal with custody of the children, you are sufficiently psyched up to put through your case and put in the fight, but also be mentally prepared that you might lose the plot for full custody. Whether or not you believe you did more for the children or that you had been a better *mother* to them than she was, is not relevant here – it is simply, in my view, the age-old conventional belief that mothers are naturally better suited for the home and nurturing of children, and fathers, for provision, and protection. These principles are entrenched in most national family laws and, in some cases, indiscriminately and mindlessly.

Today, it is possible that men and women are equally matched for traditionally nurturing roles. What concerns me as a member of modern society, however, is that the world calls for equality between genders, and I subscribe to that 100 percent. I also subscribe to one of the truths on which that call stands: women today can do just about anything men do and vice versa. But when it comes to custody issues, men face a more significant hurdle having to prove beyond reasonable expectations that they too can offer just about everything nurturing that a natural woman can for her children. I'll leave that there for you to ponder.

Psyche yourself. If you are denied custody, don't see that as a reflection of your inability to equally offer nurturing love to your children or a negation of the tremendous efforts you have already poured into them until that point – it is just how the realities of many family laws work. Sadly, when you pour everything into equally nurturing your children, you don't do so, recording and documenting every element of your input because you don't hope for a breakdown and a subsequent requirement to prove the love you've poured into your children. It doesn't make you a fool; you are a good father.

If you are reading this, a separation or divorce is probably imminent now or has already happened. Where dealing with the children is concerned, I want to share a few things that may be worth keeping in mind. It doesn't matter if you have done some things differently by the time you read this; you did your best in the circumstances. If the advice here offers a better way, correct those you can, and look for opportunities with your children in the future to counter what's already been done and done wrong. Again, the fact that you are reading this chapter, getting this book for someone, or telling a friend in a similar situation, means you are doing a lot of good for humanity. Stay positive.

I don't know how old your children were during your marital breakdown. If they are aged fifteen years or above, it doesn't make it easier on them, but at least they are at an age where some reasonable conversations can be had, and some understanding is possible on their part. If they are younger, then it's critical you understand this one thing, and if you had to exercise one last superpower of yours, then get your Ex also to understand this because if both of you do, it will be the most excellent proof of your love, individually and collectively, for your children. And this is it – *"Kids just want to be kids."*

Kids just want to be kids. I am not saying to shield them from the reality of the happenings. Still, I am saying do everything in your power to ensure that amid everything you as adults are going through, you give the kids everything they need to: *(i) continue enjoying being kids and (ii) not get burdened with becoming adults, sharing your adulthood problems, or having to also make the difficult choice between you two* – they are kids, leave them to be. Everything else outside this is a choice for you two as adults. It lessens the damage divorce does to them if you both agree on this one thing. Yes, you may have taken away one of the greatest components of a quality childhood, a home with both parents, but do everything else to help them continue enjoying their childhood. Kids just want to be kids.

From talking to many couples, there is no such thing as *"the perfect time"* to tell your children about a divorce or a breakdown. I often say to keep three things in mind – first, the earlier, the better; second, the earlier, the better; third, the earlier, the better – but only when you are both thoroughly convinced divorce is the only way to go. Believe it or not, children have some of the most amazing intuitions you can imagine, and way before you both decide to tell them about it, they have probably already picked up on the signs. They may not have asked about it for fear of upsetting you or, depending on their age, because they have no idea how to articulate the questions in their minds or because they are afraid it will turn out to be true, but children have extraordinarily sharp intuitions. You might try convincing yourself they didn't see you arguing in the bedroom or garden or going to see a counselor or that you hid your cold wars well. Listen, children don't have to see; they feel it all; they feel the vibe in the air, on your skin. They smell your pain. Children feel it all, so please, do it before it becomes too obvious to hide, do it before they ask questions, and do it before one of you leaves home abruptly.

Ideally, do it together. And if they have a grandma, grandpa, aunties, or uncles they love who understand the psychological needs of the situation and are willing to sit with you both to speak to the children – even better. It offers them a cushion or layer of emotional safety. That's because, believe it or not, when breaking the news to them, some children may interpret it as pressure on them to choose between either parent. Having a neutral person there, who they know loves them too, takes that unnecessary burden off them until they can better digest it all.

In deciding to tell your children about the breakdown, optics are critical. I know you want to tear each other's throats out, but for your children, the optics will communicate more than what you actually say in words. Sit together. Get the frowns off your faces. Keep the tone low and warm. For those fifteen or sixty minutes, show the children they still have parents, NOT warlords. Hug them individually and hug them together after the conversation. Please, psyche yourselves before the meeting and play your part for the children. If there is one sacrifice you should be willing to make for your children, this is probably one.

It's one thing to try letting them know that they still have parents they can count on as pillars, but it is another thing altogether if they sense that the people they thought were loving parents are two strangers they hardly know. You need to help them walk away with the picture that they will still have a team they can count on – that is instructive. Between yourselves, you may have decided to stop being a team for each other, but that was your adult decision. Where the children are concerned, you are still their team, and FOR THEM, you must be that team when they need you to be. Fight all you can with yourselves after that. I am sharing lessons from mistakes I would never want you to make, not even if you were my worst enemy. The children must not be shortchanged for decisions they never made.

What I find more critical when engaging the children after a breakdown is what you say to them. I may not be the world's most outstanding expert, but I have been through the rungs and seen breakdowns that worked well and some that didn't. I think I have seen enough to offer five key insights briefly. It doesn't mean these are the only things you should say to your children during those heavy conversations. I am merely suggesting that you consider incorporating them into the essential things you communicate to them.

First and foremost, children, irrespective of their ages, must be assured that no ongoing breakdown is their fault, especially if they are younger than fifteen. Please don't say, *"But why would they even get that idea? None of us has told them or accused them of such."* It is a child thing; it isn't about you. Just as you may have pondered scenarios about what it was you did or missed to get things where they are, children do so too, and one of the most common things they assume is, *"What if mom and dad were happy together with no problems until I was born?"* Yes, many children I have encountered in these circumstances think this. They may not articulate it as I have or even voice it out. But by talking to them, you'll know it is there. It doesn't make sense, doesn't make adult logic, but it is *their reality*, and you don't have to understand or live their existence to address it, so do something about it – let them know lovingly that the break-up is not their fault.

It will hardly cross your mind in the heat of the break-down because we think children think like us, but most children silently go through life immediately after the collapse, thinking the mess was their fault. You don't have to be a child to know that it is such a heavy and unnecessary burden for them to carry. The assurance must come from both parents. If you can convince your Ex that you both need to assure the children that none of what you are dealing with is their fault, great! If you cannot, still do your part – it helps lift their invisible yet real burden.

Second. Without a doubt, the greatest need of a child from both parents is love. As they face the burdensome reality that they will be losing you being together, it is also essential to make them aware that they will not be losing your love. *"You always have, you still do, and you will forever love them"* is the message to deliver, not once, not twice, not thrice, but as many times as you get the op-portunity until *"the new life"* gets somewhat normalized, albeit it never entirely does.

Understand, your children never experienced you lov-ing them before your marriage to your partner. When your children were born, you were already together *(at least, this is the most logical scenario)*. *So,* they automatically associate the parental love they get from each or both of you with you being together. As such, when a breakup or divorce happens, the big question in their minds is,

"Will the love I get from Daddy break down too, now that the unified source of that love is broken down?" So please, be sincere with them — assure them that however often and in whatever way you have loved them, it will not change.

When my breakdown first happened, my kids were taken away. After that, it took a year of battling in court to get to see them, and when I finally did, I had a few things I wanted so badly to share with them. Before this point, the kids had not been blind, they saw everything I was subjected to, but it was still partly my duty to preserve the sanctity of their relationship with both parents, which is the third consideration I want to share with you. Nobody is bad. Neither mommy nor daddy is a bad person because they are walking out of a marriage. Hold your horses under this caution — it is not your job to paint your Ex-partner as bad or evil to your children. You can do what is necessary to protect them, but you must not feed them with anger and bitterness. You may have had issues with your Ex, but the children have no altercation with their mother. Control yourself from distorting their image of her. Trust me, if there are things the children need to see and know about your Ex, they either already know or will eventually see it for themselves.

Not everything that happens in life falls in a black-and-white zone. Many more things fall in the grey area, not black, white, yes, no, high, low, just in the middle. Many children who haven't yet reached the age where they can define and adopt their own philosophies will undoubtedly find it hard to accept that a beautiful, warm, loving, close-knit family unit can cease to be all that without it being a *"monster's"* fault, and so in their silent minds, they may be seeking to identify who the *monster* is.

But here is the bigger reason for doing this – the breakup happened between two adults, not you and the children, not your Ex and the children. The separation or divorce occurred between you and your Ex. The animosity, anger, vengeful thoughts, etc., are between two adults, and as such, there is NO reason under the canopies of heaven or hell for the children to see either parent as bad; that would be unfair to them. They should understand that they will continue to have both parents' availability and influence beyond the breakup. Even if you think your Ex is a witch - the children need both of you to have complete childhood experiences. Yes, I understand that in most circumstances, one parent takes the children and moves away, but hopefully, this will clarify why your children need both parents for full, proper development. Remember, two adults have a problem, not the kids, so trying to score points with the kids by painting the other party black in their eyes will only end up hurting the one person you thought you were protecting – the children.

Finally, you *(both)* must assure your children that they still have you as *(i.e., you will still be)* their father and mother. Just like reassuring them of your love, in your children's minds, your fatherhood is strongly linked to you two being a couple. You will have to help them understand that being a husband to your Ex is separate from being a father to them, that you will forever be a father to them, and that everything you did for them, with them, and that they expect from you as a father will remain the same.

When Jason and Faith's marriage broke down, I already had very close ties to them and their kids. I offered, and they agreed to have the kids stay with me for a few weeks in the heat of the collapsing marriage. I think they did the right thing. Subsequently, when it was time to break the news to Analisa and Manfred *(the children)*, Faith requested I do it with them, to which I obliged, under one condition – that throughout the *"conversation"* process, they would take themselves and their animosity out of the equation for that one hour and put the kids first. They would sit together and speak slowly, reassuringly, and warmly through all the topics listed. It was in that engagement that Manfred first asked the question, and as harmless and cute as it sounded, it was a deep spot in the entire conversation. Manfred's question was this – *"If daddy and mommy won't be together, will daddy still be my daddy?"* It broke me in pieces but was also a big learning point. Since then, I have encountered either the same questions or similar thought patterns in the kids of my friends and friends of my friends who went through a divorce or breakup. You must assure them you will remain their father *(and mother)* whether they ask or not.

Let me end with this. If it turns out that as part of your divorce arrangements, your children must live for the most part with your Ex-partner, make sure you do everything possible to remain an equal influence in their lives, even if it is only through allowed phone calls weekly. No matter how resourceful a woman may be, there are some things only a man's influence can instill in a child.

If they turn out well, it will be because you continued actively being in their world and lives. Please do it for them. Yes, it may come at the price of swallowing some of your pride and occasionally accepting a certain level of arm-twisting. Still, for the sake of your kids, it is worth it – just don't succumb to being emotionally, financially, or in any other way blackmailed. That you must not accept, and my reason is simple – if your children are used against you, it is just a matter of time; you will be used against them. Yes, you may come across as heartless, but that's what a father's heart sometimes looks like.

I usually have a simple principle that has worked for me – any disagreement with my Ex concerning our kids that I consider will not affect the destinies and prospects of our children, she is allowed to win. I will state my position, but you certainly won't get a full-blown debate from me. If I am convinced, after considerations and consultations, that the matter at hand will not end well for the present prospects, livelihoods, or well-being *(physical, social, spiritual, and emotional)* of our children, I guarantee you; I'll fight it to the end. I am a father, their protector, separated or not. Always.

I want you to take just two things away from this chapter:

Firstly, *kids want to be kids; let them be.*

Secondly, tell them that nothing is their fault; you will always be their father, and they will always be loved.

CHAPTER SIX

AFTER HURRICANE EX: THE REALITY CHECK

At some point in the journey, when court, custody or family tribunal, or negotiations have resulted in a solution where parties are willing to settle to go their separate ways, you will feel some calm – partly from seeing an end in sight, partly because you are just tired from going through the extended emotional cycles, and partly because, believe it or not, you have become used to the pain and realities associated with separation. Suppose yours was a particularly brutal, vindictive, or painful separation. In that case, you may feel a cloudy but necessary shade of happiness knowing that you escaped being trapped in your relationship beyond what you had already endured. You may even be tempted to ask the forbidden question: *"How the heck did I stay in it for this long?"* Shake it off; you weren't hypnotized – you just understood life a little differently. Now, after this experience, you have had the chance to understand life even more differently than before.

In this seeming state of *the calm after the storm*, when hopefully your brain has taken back control from your heart, there are certain realities I want to share with you that you need to embrace, realities you may not necessarily like. I didn't want to accept some at first, too, for years. Nevertheless, these realities are genuine and, when taken, place you in better stead to reshape and reinvent your future – *the future after the storm*.

Talking about storms, my friends and I like to picture them as personalized hurricane situations – our respective divorces. It usually comes unexpectedly and blows many things down with the feeling of terror and the pain of loss. But after the storm blows over, you have to face the painful reality that your home, or part of it, ceases to exist, your neighborhood has been hard hit, and you have to decide whether to move away or stay and rebuild and if it is the latter, then, to rebuild in a manner that makes you resilient and ready to face any similar or worse storms in the future. How much of these realities you know and embrace determines how resilient and better you live after the hurricane – your hurricane. In the case of my friend Joshua, it was *Hurricane Goldie*; for Tim, it was *Hurricane Bertha*; for Brandon, *Hurricane Madjoa*; for Stephen, *Hurricane Biola*; for Kagwe, it was *Hurricane Akello*; for you, it may have been *Hurricane…*

First reality check, stop wishing her evil, bro – it won't make your life better, and 99.9 percent of the time, what you wish her won't happen. Yes, the pain may not entirely vanish; yes, the memories will flash back now and again; yes, you may see how the kids are being managed and say, *"That's not how I would have wanted it done,"* yes, you may think she put you through hell and seemed to have gotten away with it unpunished. Yes, you may feel justice was not correctly served, but listen, you could equally channel all that energy into something useful that helps you get back on your feet, bigger and better. Besides, the world doesn't run on your *"bad wishes"* for fuel. STOP wishing her evil. Vengeance is bad energy; bad energy is depleting, and the more you produce, the more she wins, even after she is gone. My friend Kojo captures it better – he says, *"It is like letting someone else live in your head or heart without paying rent."* Or, as I heard someone else once say, *"It is like eating poison and hoping that she dies instead."* Wake up to the reality, gentlemen – she's gone; get her out of your mind too. It may be challenging and lengthy, but not doing it will hurt you more. Get her out of your system, and NO, the way around that is not to jump into another relationship immediately because you will hurt someone else until you purge your system of any residual bitterness. Believe me, it's true what they say, "*Hurt people, only hurt other people.*" Let it go. But beyond that, we all attract the energies we radiate, so walking around with the energy that wants to hurt someone will only attract you to someone whose energy is seeking to be hurt. It is not worth it.

Many years after Danny and his Ex, Natasha, married, he started feeling like he was being punished for something he never did. So, during one of their pillow-talk sessions, he made Natasha aware that she sometimes treated him as though he was being punished for a wrong someone else did to her but whom she could not. She denied it. Eventually, it ruined them, and much later, after their divorce, Danny found out she had sadly been a victim of some childhood abuse from her very first boyfriend but had never healed from it. Your untamed and unpurged hurt will only make you hurt someone else. Get help if you are still bitter, face your demons, give it enough time, and purge it – it will make life bigger, better, and brighter. Let it go. I need you; the brotherhood of men needs you too.

Reality check number two, you are NOT your Ex's defense lawyer, so stop acting like one. You may have been physically separated, but you need to ask yourself and answer truthfully – are you emotionally and mentally detached too? If you are not, the tendency is that when her name comes up, you will still likely be in "*husband mode,*" either trying to speak for, defend, or shield her. It would be best if you consciously started learning to catch yourself doing it. You are not, were not, and cannot now be responsible for her present, past, and future actions. It may be cute, but it damages your recovery and ability to move on. Otherwise, maybe, just maybe, you shouldn't have separated in the first place, and perhaps, you need to think it all through again. I am not an advocate for divorce, but once you get to the point that it is the only option for both of you, be committed to becoming a better man, including not taking responsibility for your Ex's actions, utterances, behavior, nothing. You are not her *defense attorney*.

Third reality check – you are divorced, check! You are physically separated, check! You have successfully disconnected emotionally and mentally, check! Hoorah! But, if you have children together, or property or a business that requires both your inputs – she will still be a part of your world, the life of your kids, business, and partnerships. Bro, you need to be clear about this one thing – she is only a part of your world, just like everyone else, not a part of your life. Any treatment beyond what is regular towards everyone else should be premised entirely on what additional benefits it yields to your children and your common businesses and assets. No one is asking you to be unnecessarily inhumane, rude, or dismissive towards your Ex, no. After all, she is still the mother of your children, and insofar as it helps the children still enjoy the blessings of having a mother and a father, it should be enough. That's where it ends. Please stop the *almost-intimate* treatments you give her, the gifts, dates that you spuriously refer to as *"just-catch-*

ing-up meetings," and everything else you will only do for a woman in your life, a woman you are in love with. Unless, of course, you still are — and that's *not necessarily bad.* But if you intend to move on, she must remain in your world, not your life.

You can no longer be responsible for her personal choices and consequences, nor clean up after her actions if reckless. Be good to her, as you would anyone else, but understand she is only still part of your world - not your life. It is this understanding that most friends and family don't get during a divorce or breakup process. For them, the feeling is, *"If you can delete her out of your life and have nothing to do with her ever again, you will be fine"* — well, it doesn't quite work out as black and white as that, bro. No more a part of your life, yes, no more a part of your world, no. You cannot just pretend and wish her away. She is there and human; sometimes, you will need her for the kids — it just cannot be like before. You must accept that her place and status in your world is no more what it used to be — your children are both in your life and world, your Ex, only in your world. Your siblings and parents are in your life and world; your Ex is only in your world. You understand, right?

Reality four. From now on, you will need some ground rules to function in your newfound worlds of *no longer being together.* And that means ground rules around visits, finances, the children, and even how you relate to shared friends. My only key points in setting up or dealing with these ground rules are one, you will have to accept some of their conditions, just as you expect her to take some of yours. Second, your focus should not be on your rights or your logic here – it should be about whether you can achieve some progress with their demands. It should be worth considering if reasonable progress can be made if nobody's (especially the children's) destiny or potential, or opportunities will be compromised by it. Sometimes that progress will be for the kids, sometimes for you and the kids, sometimes for her and the kids, and sometimes for her – insofar as it offers some over-arching progress, especially for the kids, then consider it. Third, keep the safety of the children and your peace of mind paramount in whatever you agree to.

A fifth reality check – most men have a heart for their kids, and I have no doubt you do too. If you do, chances are that what your Ex can no longer get out of you be-cause of the dissolution or breakup, she may try getting by using the kids. Warning: don't start getting paranoid; not all women do this. You knew your Ex before the split; if she could do this, there is a high chance you would have known before the break. Whatever happens, DON'T allow your kids to be used against you. Else, it is just a matter of time before you will be used against them. Once it starts, once you yield, once you let it fes-ter, it won't stop. So, don't let it. Yes, sometimes it will come across as though you are heartless – but some-times, that's what it takes to protect your children and your peace of mind.

When Charles and his ex, Deborah, split up, sever-al times he paid for holidays and events he knew the kids would love, and Deborah would only cash them in or sometimes let the tickets go to waste. Months later, Charles found out the kids were never actually being taken on the breaks he had been paying for and that several demands made on behalf of the kids, who lived with Deborah, were a cashing scheme. He stopped and, being a banker, had an account opened for his eldest daughter, which he funded minimally. He further paid vendors directly for services the children needed, which were only requested now by the kids. It got Deborah furious for months on end. But it was the right thing to do. He was responsible for his children, not for Deborah.

Reality check number six — stop lying to yourself about love. It isn't true that you will NEVER love again. I vowed this vehemently, too, after my split. Often, when friends and family would say, *"Oh, you are still young; you cannot stay single forever,"* I would kiss my teeth, shake my head, and retort, *"Never again."* That was just the pain talking. You have been hurt; the wounds are still raw and bleeding; anything that looks like what started the bleeding, you will resist vehemently. It is normal to feel that way. But heal first and heal properly. And when you have healed and found yourself, often, love may find you.

This leads me to believe that when you take your time to become the best version of yourself, someone who even you would like to fall in love with, you are most likely to attract the right person to fall in love with you. I joke sometimes; just be wise to walk in love and not fall in love this time. Besides, there is a positive side to all that — after everything you have been through, you won't be going into another relationship starting from scratch; you will be starting from experience. Now you know what questions to ask, what stones not to leave unturned, now you know you are responsible for your happiness, now you know yourself enough to understand who is compatible and who isn't, now you know that a relationship will only last as long as there is something long-lasting you both want out of it, now you know what is fleeting and what are enduring expectations to have of each other. I often say that where you are or have been on your life journey before meeting someone plays a big role in determining how successful that relationship will go. Some people cross paths when they have matured in matters of the heart and have experienced what works for them and what doesn't. Some meet at points in their lives when neither have learned any lessons nor found the versions of themselves that they will happily fall in love with.

If it does happen to you again, though - *love, I mean* - I am shamelessly happy for you, but PLEASE, heal first. It took me a little over two years to purge and heal. It may take you seven, maybe one, maybe months, but however long it takes, please – heal properly first.

And when love does find you this time, I have only one piece of advice I want you to consider – don't see the next woman as your Ex. She is not. If you catch yourself always seeing your Ex in her, making comparisons, or drawing similarities, you will have ruined it before it started. You are most likely never adequately healed. Don't brush it aside. Step back; heal first. Otherwise, your next fall, if it does happen, will be more devastating. Heal first, then love again - if it finds you.

Live with the mindset that love can happen again, BUT you won't force it to hurry. Until it finds you, live a day at a time, and focus on making yourself a better, more peaceful, happier man. You might be wondering: did Kodi find love again? Well, I mean… you know… thing is… quite frankly… errrrrr

Let me leave you with this anonymous quote; maybe it will inspire you:

"Love is not something you go out looking for. Love finds you, and when it does, ready or not, it'll be the best thing to ever happen to you."

CHAPTER
SEVEN

REINVENT YOURSELF

One of the best advice I got when I divorced was – *"now you need to focus on reinventing yourself."* At the time, I didn't even know what that meant. It took me over two years after receiving that advice to grasp it fully – I hope yours takes a shorter time.

None of us became the current version of ourselves overnight. Some of our personalities, behaviors, orientations, and world views today were formed over days, weeks, months, and years. The thing is, our minds barely keep track of which ones developed over what timeframe; after all, that's not knowledge we need to get through our daily routines of living, so it is certainly not one the brain keeps track of prudently. However, if something like a habit or a mindset takes longer to form, you can only reasonably expect it wouldn't take days to *"un-form."*

When you think about reinventing yourself after becoming a divorcee, don't think about it like your whole life has to change; no, that will overwhelm and stress you out. You only need to change certain aspects or do certain things differently that were previously necessary because you were married but which are now somewhat redundant. I know it sounds cliché, but it will surprise you that without conscious effort to recalibrate our minds, many divorcees go through the rest of their lives still subconsciously living out certain parts of their routines and thought processes as though they were still married. If you think about it, it's why the brain helps form habits, right? It recognizes your new circumstance, e.g., you are newly married, it notices the actions, thinking, and behaviors that have become routine because of your unique circumstances, and in order not to waste your thinking energy on those regularized behaviors, it automates those actions, thoughts, and behaviors – we call them habits. The problem, however, is that once they are automated, the mind doesn't suddenly de-automate them as soon as you become a divorcee; that only happens when you consciously determine what actions, thoughts, and behaviors are no longer relevant to your divorcee status and STOP playing them out. It must be conscious.

Here is a good one. Once they get married, most men stop trying to stay personally happy. We may not necessarily think it is the job of our wives to make us happy; no, we just tend to make our happiness a minimal priority. If you hear most men in marriage speak, their focus is evidently about *"doing all they can to make their FAMILY happy"* – except that *"family,"* in their subconscious mind, doesn't include them. And it isn't good. How can you genuinely be joyful towards others when you are unhappy yourself? No man can give what he does not have, including happiness. Most men, when trying to justify their lack of self-care, will say things like *"I am happy when my family is happy"* – that, my friend, is a lie manufactured from hell's laundry room. I share these things so that hopefully, you can first claw back some of the joys you have missed out on, in the name of being a husband, joys that you are entitled to, and second, so that if you hopefully do marry again, you see and do things differently.

Learn to be happy by yourself. Learn to be happy for *you.* Learn to be happy with yourself. This is the biggest reinvention project you are going to embark on. If you do, and you must, it will have a tremendous effect on your life and living it more profoundly, more beautifully.

If you can learn to be happy for yourself, you will carry your happiness wherever you go and find it easier being happy, irrespective of WHO you are with or without. It must be conscious; you must embrace the truth that you deserve to be always happy – it depends on you. There are so many ways of going about it, but I will share a few obvious ones and hope they inspire you to think up others. *(You should consider getting my other book, 'The Manifesto of Living' and go straight to chapter 6 titled, 'Live to Die, Don't Die to Live' – it will be a fulfilling read and real value for money, believe me)*

Before I got divorced, I used to work hard to make sure my family had a holiday every year, and for the most part, it was to places I felt the "*family*" might find beneficial; for example, it had to be child friendly, it had to have experiences the children would love, it had to be a place where the children could get some level of professional supervision, so my wife could take needed rest. It wasn't necessarily where I fancied going if *I* was given the option. And for the first few years after my separation, guilt kept me from going on any holiday. Yeah, I was feeling bad that I was going on a holiday when I wasn't sure if "*my family would too,*" or even if they did, how it would be without me to take care of the logistics, as I usually would - until I snapped out of it.

I, too, deserved to be happy by myself. So, I took a trip to some places I had always wanted to visit, for me, by me, with me. I went to Greece, Germany, and the Dubai desert, among other places, and not only did I travel, I did some of what I had always wanted to do for me – I did a bungee jump, a skydive, and a sports car race – I am not an adrenaline junkie, but these were the very things our minds, and sometimes our wives tell us we cannot do because, "*You know you are a married man; you cannot just do anything, right?*" or "*What if something happens to you, are you thinking about your family?*" Believe it or not, there is a thin line between needing to be a responsible family man and stopping to live, and if you aren't very strong-minded and conscious about your happiness, you most likely will stop living.

My advice to all men, divorced or not, is this – find three things that make you happy consistently, three things that, every time you indulge, you derive pleasantness and joy, and three things that your pleasure from indulgence will hardly diminish. Then, do them often, maybe once a month or even every week. I love reggae; I love movies; I love swimming; I love exploring seafood; I love traveling and road trips, and I love being in company that allows me to laugh annoyingly loud and hard. My joy multiplies rather than diminishes when I engage in these things, so I do at least two every week. Please, you deserve to be happy – find a few things that bring you joy and do them regularly. Your happiness is your responsibility; in fact, it is the first thing you owe to yourself – do it for you.

Next, I suggest you find impactful ways to add value to yourself. I mean, you are divorced now. The future has always been there, waiting for you, but you probably have one less pressure on your finances or time, and you might as well use it to add some value to yourself – it is the only way you are going to be ready for the future when you meet it, and it will come, guaranteed.

Usually, when I talk to men about adding value, the first notion that comes to them is – enhancing their careers. No. You see, that is a mental reinvention you need too. From here onward, you must think about yourself as a wholesome human; you are not only made up of your career, and you were never just a husband; you are you, and that is the most important job of all and one you should continually add value to. You are so many other things besides work and family.

Here is what I do and what I suggest. Every year, I do my best to take at least three courses or programs or activities, and the variety is wide and readily available these days. One program in the year is always geared toward improving my career's relevance for the future. Effectively, I try to gauge where my profession or industry is evolving towards, what new skills will be required to remain relevant in the next one to five years, what new ideas are trending and which will become mainstream in that timeframe, what new ways of doing existing professional tasks will make me professionally more efficient and cutting edge. Once I find something that meets my criteria, I sign up. It could even be something that may help you make a career change, assuming there's a new career path you had meant to explore while you were married but couldn't make the time to explore due to *"family commitments."* Now is a perfect time.

I choose something that improves my life skills for one of the other two programs each year. For example, this year, I took an advanced swimming program taught by the military. It was cool learning new tricks used by an elite survival swimmer. For lack of a better phrase, the experience made me feel… *more*. It could be that you already know how to cook and want to improve your cooking, language, networking, or driving skills…. Improve something you already know about but isn't directly career-related – something that makes you a better part of society or your immediate world.

And, of course, lastly, do something entirely new – not a career or social skill – something just for the experience. I, for example, am learning how to ride a motorbike and make chocolates this year. I have never done either before, and I do not intend to become a grand prix racer or a resident Marriot hotel chocolatier – I am doing it because that's how we live - by adding new experiences to our lives consistently. Next year, I plan a scuba dive and another bungee jump with my two nieces and eldest daughter. If you don't look for new experiences and improve yourself, believe me, you have stopped living – in marriage or outside it. You need to indulge in fresh, healthy, and exciting experiences constantly. So, live. *(Now I think you ought to read chapter 6 of 'The Manifesto of Living')*

Finally, one of the reinventions of yourself that I believe will be super useful for life beyond marriage, or even "*life in marriage again*," is connections. Most men, including myself, once they enter marriage, seem to take on the posture automatically: *it is me and my 'family' now.*

Gradually, without taking notice, you drift away from networks and people – you become isolated and eventually trapped in your marriage. The trapping tends to happen because once you have been isolated long enough, you soon regrettably realize you don't have many people to reach out to, even when you need help, so you convince yourself, "*Well, at least my family is here for me.*" Listen, bro, NO human being was created to be isolated, it is just not in our wiring, and you must fight everything that seeks to isolate you.

If your spouse, for any reason, thought, complained or kicked against you remaining plugged into your networks while you were married – that was not you; that was her insecurity. Never marry insecurity – it will always paint your opportunities with its fears, which is not a healthy environment. Our successes, our growth, and our general progress in life *(and, for that matter, the benefits they accrue to our families)* are directly linked to the number and quality of networks we are plugged into, and no marriage has the right to truncate that lifeline. None.

But now you are divorced. Yes, getting back into some networks will look like, "*Aaah, you are only back now because your marriage didn't work, huh?*" Believe me, self-inflicted or actual jabs like this from friends and colleagues are a tiny price to pay to get re-plugged into humanity *(networks)*. You need it. We all do.

One of the many things I had to give up as a married man was my membership in an elite fraternity. Even though looking back now, I still cannot find a logical reason for agreeing to step out of it in the first place,

I am simply happy and fulfilled being welcomed back many years later. Plugging yourself back into sound and worthwhile networks as part of your reinvention process is helpful on many levels. Still, most importantly, each human being represented in your network is a doorway to an opportunity or several opportunities. But it isn't just that; it offers you an escape from isolation and forces you to escape your previous mindset of pretending to be *"unavailable,"* all in the name of being a family man. That is a balance every family man needs to find - to draw quality energy, inspiration, and opportunities from his networks to pour back into his family.

Reinventing yourself is something you must do for yourself.

If you have never heard the Biblical parable of the prodigal son, you should go check it out in the book of *Luke, chapter fifteen.* Most of us divorcees are by ourselves, both the prodigal son and the father of the prodigal son in that story. We must both forgive ourselves as the father did forgive his son and reinvent ourselves, just as the son, on returning, had to agree to change from the rags he wore to decent clothing. Reinventing yourself is what you do to appreciate that *"you found your once-lost self"* – just as the father was thankful for finding his lost son. And if for nothing at all, for those whose separation came with losing regular direct contact with their young children, listen to me – reinventing yourself is needed to guarantee that you are a better version of yourself when your children come back to meet you. And they will come back one way or another.

So, go out there and reinvent yourself in whatever number of ways you must – have no regrets, and be proud of what you accomplished in marriage, no matter how short or long it lasted. You just had one more experience to add to life's resume. Polish it, groom up and dress up *(reinvent)* and present yourself for life's most prominent job yet – *the job of living.*

IN CONCLUSION, STAY TRUE TO THE BROTHERHOOD

Whether you like it or not, you are a veteran now. You have had a taste of a pill many people haven't. As I said, these experiences have no winners, but at least you know more than many men what to do differently.

For one, avoid getting entangled in a relationship where you constantly have to receive much less than what you are giving and willing to give. Eventually, it will drain you, wear you and burn you out. Relationships are not supposed to be a one-way street. Beyond agreeing to add value to each other, be each other's inspiration to grow, and be an excellent ecosystem for young humans to be raised – everything else takes work, and I mean work from both partners. And may I add - *selfless work*. It cannot be a partnership in which everyone gives *"fifty-fif-ty"* – no, everyone must give 100 percent of themselves at every point. So, make that your standard going for-ward – you cannot be in anything akin to a relationship in which you are the only one giving value or in which you are consistently getting significantly less than you are putting in.

Based on all you may have experienced now, do what is legally necessary in the future to protect yourself. For example, I have decided not to go into another deep relationship without a prenuptial agreement should it end in marriage. No, you are not being faithless in your new partner or being selfish or untrusting of her. On the contrary, you are the only person in this world who genuinely has your interest and whom you can 100 percent trust. You owe it to yourself to protect yourself. No one else will, which is the sad reality of our world today. Some folks have told me they will go the *"Hakimi way"* in any future marital endeavor. I laugh both in excitement but also on caution. In case you haven't caught on yet, the *Hakimi way* refers to a social media viral article about Achraf Hakimi Mouh, a Moroccan professional footballer who plays for Ligue 1 club Paris Saint-Germain and who is purported to have been involved in a divorce case initiated by his wife, seeking more than 50 percent of his wealth. The report states that the wife was stunned in court to find out her footballer husband had no wealth to his name and, by extension – nothing to be sued for. He previously transferred all his wealth into his mother's name. The news got men around the world super excited. Let me confess now – I was, too, to some extent. I cannot vouch for how true the story is, but it is the principle that matters – he protected himself. A word of caution about the Hakimi way, though – not every mother is an angel. Sometimes, you may find your partner is an excellent help than your mother or both are. All

I will say is this – know who you are dealing with. It is not the only way. I know men who have gone to great lengths – some have had their weddings in particular jurisdictions that have favorably automatic divorce laws, some have ensured most of their wealth was held under offshore trusts, companies, and the like, and some have signed up very complex prenuptial agreements, the list is indeed endless, but I think you get the drift – protect yourself first. See it as wearing a helmet before getting on the marriage speed bike. Get professional advice on what works, but then again, be reasonable in the extent to which you go; otherwise, you could equally end up burning an excellent woman to protect yourself against bad women. Be smart but be human too. Find the right balance.

Finally, let me say this – please, stay true to the brotherhood of men. It is a critical appeal I am making to you and all men. Many men go through invested relationship breakups, breakdowns, and divorces painfully, quietly, and in most cases, ashamed or scared to talk about it for fear that society will see them as weak. It is a reality I am sure you also may have experienced. The point I wish to make is simply this – when you see, hear, or know another man going through breakdowns of relationships they have emotionally, physically, and financially invested in – reach out to them and offer a helping hand. Sometimes it may just be an ear another brother needs to pour out his pain or frustration, sometimes a non-judgmental space to help them find their peace of mind or regain their waning strength; sometimes, it may be someone holding their hands and sharing a word of prayer with them.

In whatever way you can help, help a brother out there. The help could even be as simple as buying them a copy of this book to read too. But listen, bro – we must be each other's keeper. Good men get burned all the time, mostly not out of choice, and it will take other men to raise them as kings again.

What can I say? I wish you and every man out there with some good left in them the best this life offers.

All the very best; I love you all.

PLEASE...

First, thank you sincerely for making the time to read my book. It is okay if you and I disagree on some points – it is a good thing. But if this book made you ask questions, got you to consider different perspectives on issues, or gave you a reason to reaffirm beliefs you already held, then I suppose it is fair to say it has been worth the read. If so, I count on your good nature and kindness to recommend it or buy a copy for friends, family, or colleagues. And if it is not too much to ask, leave it a helpful review here on Amazon so that others can find and read it too - it only takes a few minutes. I also have a landing page at www.kodiblackmanbooks.com where you can interact with me or share experiences that can enrich the lives of others. Thank you for everything.

OTHER BOOKS BY KODI BLACKMAN

TITLE:	**WHEN GOOD MEN GET BURNED**
SUBTITLE:	How to Cope and Reinvent Yourself as A Divorcee
AUTHOR:	Kodi BLACKMAN
SUMMARY:	If you are a good man faced with divorce or a breakdown of an invested relationship, chances are you will feel like it is you against the world, drowned in a sea of mixed emotions, or plain angry. You will repeatedly replay the last memories, trying to pinpoint what went wrong. Believe me; you are normal and not alone, I assure you. This book is a support system for men who have gone or are going through a divorce, and it is by someone who has been through it. But Kodi goes beyond your emotions. He shares tips for managing the extended family to ensure their desire to protect your interests does not create chaos. He passionately shares how to calm your young children so they do not feel unnecessarily burdened in the aftermath of a split. He concludes with great advice on setting boundaries with your Ex and, more importantly, how to re-invent yourself into becoming a better man. Men hardly get this invaluable support – I hope they find it in this book.

TITLE: **THE MANIFESTO OF LIVING**

SUBTITLE: Living Life to The Full, In Freedom, In Wealth

AUTHOR: Kodi BLACKMAN

SUMMARY: Although the book's size is misleading, its simplicity is captivating, and its content, generational. These six short revealing chapters will help you build a mentality that defies every challenge life will throw at you, ground your children in wealth even before they are born, and reshape your understanding of other freedoms *(beyond financial freedom)* you will need to live your best and fullest life. It further offers you practical insights into the real power of connectedness. But that is not all – you might be surprised to discover that what you thought was *reality* may be one-half of a *bigger reality*. I can guarantee you will enjoy this book and leave with a new or unfamiliar perspective on some aspects of living.

TITLE: **MAKE AI JOBLESS, PROTECT YOUR CAREER**

SUBTITLE: A Simple Guide to Protecting Your Career from AI and Emerging Technologies

AUTHOR: Kodi BLACKMAN

SUMMARY: AI is here – is your career future-proofed? There has been much talk about Artificial Intelligence *(AI)*, emerging technologies, and their unlimited capabilities. If you are not a *"Techie,"* you will be frightened by the question, *"Will AI replace your career?"* Here is the truth – every career has an aspect that can and will be replaced by AI and other new technologies. As the replacement becomes more frequent, so will your need to remain relevant. Should that scare you? Well, not if you have future-proofed your career. That's what this book gives you – an understanding of what the threats are across several industries, insights into what skills to develop to future-proof your career, how to stand out in a crowded job market, how to leverage AI and other technologies to your benefit, and how best to prepare for the unknown future changes in the job market.

TITLE: **2045 – THE YEAR AFRICA CONQUERS THE WORLD**

SUBTITLE: Why Africa Will Be a Powerhouse in Two Decades

AUTHOR: Kodi BLACKMAN

SUMMARY: Africa is surrounded by so much negativity that even Africans themselves believe there is no hope. That was what I thought too. When one starts to examine the slow but growing facts and numbers surrounding the ongoing marriage between education and technology across Africa, the impacts of brain gain from Africa's diaspora, shifts in political and economic power from West to East, their impact on Africa's global reorientation, and Africa's journey towards becoming the most youthful, fertile and likely most populated continent in the world– suddenly if you put it all together, it doesn't look like a continent of gloom and doom anymore, but of immense prospects. This book explores five significant trends that leave Africa no choice but to become a political and economic powerhouse in just two decades if…

TITLE:	**HERE IS YOUR TICKET; COME TO AFRICA**
SUBTITLE:	9 Secrets to Successfully Do Business and Diplomacy in Africa
AUTHOR:	Kodi BLACKMAN
SUMMARY:	There are reasons you cannot do business in Africa the same way you would in America, Europe, and Asia. This book is a straightforward guide to successfully doing business and diplomacy in Africa. It explores everything from the influence of culture and tradition on business behaviors, the personal nature of doing business, the absurd complexity of its politics, local economic nuances, and more. To a Westerner or persons from other cultures, it is easy to get overwhelmed and frustrated with how things work in Africa. In this book, Kodi Blackman declutters the frustration by helping you understand the basis for the behaviors and nuances. More importantly, he shares cultural basics to master, safely playing politics without being in politics, reading the local economies, and more. This book is essential reading for you, your team, or anyone intending to travel to Africa.

TITLE:	**GOD VERSUS AI**
SUBTITLE:	How AI and Emerging Technologies May Affect Our Relationship with God
AUTHOR:	Kodi BLACKMAN
SUMMARY:	Technology today is almost *omnipresent* – it is everywhere and in everything we do; almost *omnificent* - unlimited in creative power; and with the scary pace at which AI and Machine Learning are developing and refining, technology is practically omniscient - all-knowing *(okay, a bit far-fetched, maybe)*. Still, technology is marching towards Omni status faster than most humans. With all these developments, it is easy to see why some boldly think technology, especially AI, is some manifest god. That is not the debate of this book. This book explores the intersections between religion and technology, the rise of Artificial Intelligence, the future of religion in an AI world, AI, the search for meaning, and finally, the relationship between AI and God. At the end of it, hopefully, you can ask yourself the question, *"Is God manifesting through technology?"*

TITLE: **MEN ARE TIRED BEING MEN**

SUBTITLE: Helping Men Be the Humans Society Forbids Them to Be

AUTHOR: Kodi BLACKMAN

SUMMARY: Every boy and man should read this book. It is a vital global rebellion we all need to join. Over the centuries, society and religion have made men into many things they are not. *"Men don't cry; it's a sign of weakness."* In painful circumstances, *"you must swallow the pain like a man."* In courtship, *"it is the man who should do the chasing,"* and one and one and on. In this book, Kodi Blackman questions the behavioral identities created by society for men to wear and ponders whether these identities have stripped men of their humanity. He also explores the tensions between society and nature's expectations of men and between what society frowns on about men and what men indeed could have become were it not for society's molding. This little book might be a revolutionary contribution to humanity.

9 7 9 8 3 9 9 3 8 5 1 0 5